Delicious Detox Cleanse!

<u>Detox</u>

I0417123

Easy Raw Food Recipes and Step-By-Step Plan To Cleanse Your Body For Explosive Energy, Health, And Weight Loss!

Sarah Brooks

STOP!!! Before you read any further....Would you like to know the Secrets of Body Transformation?

If your answer is yes, then you are not alone. Thousands of people are looking for the secret to rapidly burn body fat, keep the weight off, become healthier, and truly transform their body and life for good.

If you have been searching for these answers without much luck, you are in the right place!

Not only will you gain incredible insight in this book, but because I want to make sure to give you as much value as possible, right now for a limited time you can get full **100% FREE access to a VIP bonus EBook** entitled **THE 7 KEYS TO BODY TRANSFORMATION!**

Just Go Here For Free Instant Access:

www.liveFitVIP.com

Table Of Contents

Introduction

I want to thank you and congratulate you for purchasing the book, *"Detox: Delicious Detox Cleanse! – Easy Raw Food Recipes And Step-By-Step Plan To Cleanse Your Body For Explosive Energy, Health, And Weight Loss!"*

This "Detox" book contains proven steps and strategies on how to cleanse your body of harmful toxins and substances that are keeping you from performing to your full potential. Whether you want to simply cleanse your body, lose weight, have more energy, or feel stronger, detox is a great way to make you feel better every day.

Does the word 'detox' make you feel uncomfortable? Does it make you think of having to suffer through days and even weeks of extreme dieting? Is it something that you know can be good for you, but also something that you know is next to impossible to accomplish? Well, now you can change the way you think and the way you live. Detox does not have to be intimidating or nearly impossible. Learn how you can detoxify your life with natural and healthy foods that you can make every day.

More importantly, learn about the many benefits of detox and how it can help you perform better and feel better throughout the day. Aside from all the health benefits that you can get from detoxifying your body, you can also detox your way to better digestion and to rid yourself of migraines and headaches.

Finally, read on and know how you can detox your body with a step-by-step plan that you can dedicate yourself to right now.

Thanks again for purchasing this book, I hope you enjoy it!

Chapter 1: Benefits Of Detoxing

Detoxing or detoxification is a process of ridding the body of toxins and other harmful substances that have accumulated through time. Most toxins come from the food that we eat, but they can also enter the body through the air that we breathe and the medicines that we take. Regardless of how these toxins came about, they can be harmful to the body and can pose serious threats that need to be addressed if you want to stay healthy and at your peak.

Detox Benefit 1: Weight Loss

Weight loss is one of the biggest reasons why people go through detoxification, or why they even think about the idea. Detox for weight loss is fairly straightforward and easy to understand, as this involves eating natural and unprocessed foods. This means less or even no junk foods and unhealthy food options that make you put on those extra pounds. Going on a detox diet means taking in fewer calories and therefore, potentially losing weight if coupled with a good exercise program. While weight loss is perhaps the most publicized benefit of detox, most detox programs involve short-term solutions that lead to short-term results. Detox can help you lose weight, but most especially if you make it a regular part of your lifestyle.

Detox Benefit 2: Boosts Energy

Many detox programs result in increased energy levels for participating individuals. While it is hard to quantify energy or just how much of it a person has, the results pretty much speak for themselves, as people who undergo detox programs generally feel more energetic. They report feeling less sluggish and having an overall feeling of just wanting to be out and about and doing things rather than just lying around all the time. This can be attributed to the fact that detoxification releases the toxins that lower the energy levels of the body.

By steering clear of the things that provide toxins such as sugars and trans fats, the body is free from the sluggish effects of such substances. Moreover, the replacement of such negative foods with natural energy boosters such as fruits and vegetables can very much increase a person's energy levels in the best way possible. Added to this is the fact that detoxification means keeping the body hydrated at all times, resulting in more energy and better efficiency when performing daily tasks.

Detox Benefit 3: Stronger Immune System

The health benefits of detox or detoxification also include a stronger immune system. Toxins are naturally harmful for the body or at the very least, they prevent the body's systems from functioning the way that they should be. By going through cleansing programs that rid the body of these toxins, the different systems are able to function more efficiently and effectively. The immune system specifically is given a boost, allowing a person to be less prone to sicknesses and diseases once detoxification has been completed.

The removal of toxins allows the body to absorb nutrients better, including Vitamin C, which is vital for the immune system. A stronger immune system and the removal of harmful toxins and contaminants help the body fight off diseases more easily. Furthermore, detox programs make use of herbs that help the lymphatic system function better.

Chapter 2: Best Raw Food For Detoxing

Most detox programs involve a diet of raw foods. In a typical case, a raw food detox diet will have you eating at least 75 percent of raw or uncooked foods. That is, three-fourths of your diet is all about uncooked foods, as it is believed that the cooking process destroys the vitamins, minerals, and other enzymes that help in digestion and other body processes.

The good thing is that there are foods that you can eat in their raw state. In fact, the raw food detox diet is established from the idea that food is healthiest when it is eaten in its uncooked state. There are many ways for you to enjoy foods in such a manner, and these involve processes of fermenting, blending, juicing, pickling, or simply eating foods without having anything done to them. While the most common and easiest foods that you can eat as part of a raw food detox diet are fruits and certain vegetables, there are clearly raw foods that have more detox benefits than the rest.

Carrots

Carrots are among the most common foods eaten raw, and this makes them a regular part of a raw food detox diet. This root crop is famous for its Vitamin A content, which is known for promoting better eyesight. On top of this, the carrot also has a sweet flavor that makes it desirable or simply easy to consume. What many people fail to realize is that more than the benefit of the vitamins, carrots are actually a great raw food for detox because of their high fiber content. Raw carrots provide the body with a unique type of fiber that absorbs toxins and other harmful substances.

By absorbing these toxins, the fiber prevents build-up of harmful substances in the body and helps the body flush them out. Furthermore, carrots have been found to be good cleansers of estrogen, which has been related to stress. This is why women who experience pains during their menstruation period are doubly benefited with a diet of raw carrots as it eases migraines and other pains brought about by hormonal imbalance.

Try this raw detox carrot salad to cleanse your body and help balance your hormones for a more pleasurable outlook in life.

Daily Detox Carrot Salad

Ingredients:

1 medium carrot (preferable organic, unpeeled)

1 tsp. apple cider vinegar or raw coconut

1 tsp. coconut oil

½ tsp. honey (optional)

Procedure:

1. Rinse the carrot well, making sure to wash off all dirt and soil.

2. Keep the carrot unpeeled and use a grater to get long, thin, strips.

3. Rinse the carrot strips and squeeze to dry out the water.

4. In a small bowl, mix the apple cider vinegar or raw coconut with the coconut oil and season with salt. Add honey to taste if desired.

5. Drizzle the oil dressing over the carrots and toss to coat the carrots.

6. Enjoy daily!

Chapter 3: Juicing Detox Recipes

Raw foods can be good and delicious in themselves, but even the most health conscious of people will admit that eating large amount of fruits and vegetables every day can be challenging or even boring. If you want to stay true to your detox diet of eating at least eight to nine servings of fruits and vegetables daily, you should be well acquainted with the process of juicing. Juicing allows you to easily consume huge amounts of fresh and natural foods that you would otherwise find difficult to consume.

By letting foods undergo the juicing process, they turn into a liquid state that is easier to take in. Juicing also allows you to enjoy two or even more ingredients at once, making it possible to mix and match flavors according to your preference. By doing so, you not only consume more of the healthy stuff more easily, but you also get to enjoy a range of flavors that will make the detox experience a whole lot enjoyable.

Juicers are pretty easy to buy from local or online stores nowadays, and you can easily use them to juice your carrots, apples, or any fruit or vegetable you may have on hand. If you want to explore the world of juicing more, here are a few juicing detox recipes that will help you get rid of toxins and lose weight at the same time.

Apple, Carrot, and Celery Juice

Apples and carrots are some of the most common foods used for juicing. Apples naturally aid in the digestion process and help rid the body of toxins. They are also known for regulating the blood sugar levels as well as blood pressure. As for carrots, their Vitamin A and fiber content make them natural detoxifiers. Not to mention, both apples and carrots have great flavor and are easily available at any time of the year.

Ingredients:

3 pcs. apples

2 pcs. carrots

2 pcs. celery stalks

Simply chop up all of your ingredients into small and manageable pieces. You can peel the fruits and vegetables if you like, but keeping them on will retain more fiber and nutrients. Place the pieces of fruits and vegetables in the juicer a portion at a time and wait for the juice to come out. Added to the benefits of the apples and the carrots, the celery also acts as a natural diuretic that can help the body shed more fluids. This easy juicing recipe is sure to be great for detox and for weight loss as well.

Natural Protein Juice

If you want a more filling drink for your detox diet, then try this combination of almonds and sweet potatoes. This juicing recipe will provide you with your needed daily allowance of potassium and protein, and it will help you feel fueled and energized for the day ahead.

Ingredients:

1 pc. apple

½ pc. orange

1 tablespoon almonds

½ pc. sweet potato

Soak the almonds before using so that they will be easier to juice. If possible, do this a few hours before making this juice recipe. Drain the almonds from the water and put in the juicer along with the apple, half an orange, and half a sweet potato. You can also do this ahead of time and save some in the chiller so that you have your juice ready for whenever you are feeling tired.

Peach and Lychee

If you want a juicing recipe that will help you get rid of tiredness, sleepiness and overall stress, try this peach and lychee combination that will make you feel refreshed.

Ingredients:

1 pc. peach

Lychees in syrup*

½ cup coconut milk

1 tsp. honey (optional)

*as many lychees as you want

Mix one-half cup of coconut milk with one piece of peach in a juicer and as many lychees as you want. For added sweetness, mix in one teaspoon of honey as well. This drink is an excellent source of energy and will keep you hydrated throughout the day.

Chapter 4: Detox Smoothie Recipes

If you think that juicing is a great way to enjoy all those healthy fruits and vegetables, you will love smoothies even more. Smoothies are quick and easy to make and you can certainly put in any ingredient you want. Whether it's a high-fiber vegetable you want or an invigorating energy booster, you can simply mix a combination of healthy and natural foods to help get your detox going. Let your blender work on these detox smoothie recipes and you will be detoxifying, rejuvenating, and neutralizing your body in no time at all.

The Basic Detox Smoothie

Before going into some detox smoothie recipes that will help you enjoy your detox program, you should know how to make the basic detox smoothie. Instead of being a specific smoothie recipe, this basic detox smoothie will serve as a general guide. All you will need are high fiber fruits, some citrus fruits, and fibrous grains or seeds.

1. Start by selecting your high fiber fruit. Remember that this will serve as the base of your smoothie and will therefore be the main ingredient. Some of the most common fibrous fruits for detox are apples and pears, but bananas and berries are also a great choice.

2. Next, select your citrus fruit. Citrus fruits act as the main detoxifying agent as they are the ones that help clear up the digestive tract. Those that are commonly used are oranges, grapefruits and lemons. It should also be noted that most of the nutrients of these citrus fruits are present in the white meat of the peel so be sure to include them in your smoothie recipe as well.

3. Finally, add an extra kick of fiber with grains or seeds such as oatmeal, granola, or flaxseed. By adding at least a tablespoon of these fiber-rich grains and seeds, the digestive system is further cleansed, making detox and weight loss a bonus result.

4. Combine your ingredients in a blender and let it get to a smooth consistency that will make it easy to pour in a glass. You can also add a pinch of salt in the end, mixing gently with a spoon so that the saltiness will balance the flavors just right. The salt also helps in flushing out toxins and helps keep the digestive tract cleansed.

Super Green Smoothie

Green smoothies are a staple for any detox program. Just the term itself is synonymous with healthy, and they can easily make you feel better if you keep them a regular item on your menu every day. Green smoothies are those that make use of leafy greens. The dark ones particularly, like spinach and kale, are known for their rich micronutrient content. You can smoothie your way to a finely cleansed body by mixing a handful of spinach, some kale leaves and frozen berries of your choice. If you want to take the green smoothie to a whole new level, try this recipe that makes use of fourteen healthy ingredients. It may not be as easy as some smoothies are, but the benefits are definitely worth it.

Ingredients:

1 cup kale or spinach leaves

1 cup romaine lettuce leaves, torn

½ cup cucumber (chopped)

½ cup celery (chopped)

1 pc. chopped and cored pear

1 pc. chopped banana

1 cup coconut water or just water

1 tbsp. mint leaves

1 tbsp. parsley

½ pc. lemon, juiced

½ tbsp. Chia seeds

¼ inch peeled and sliced ginger root

Pinch of cinnamon (optional)

Pinch of cayenne (optional)

Pinch of turmeric (optional)

Simply place all ingredients in a blender and process until smooth. Use flavorings as desired, and sweeten with liquid stevia if preferred. Each ingredient in this super green smoothie is packed with vitamins, minerals and amino acids that help strengthen the body, fight stress and diseases and even aid in making the body look and feel better. Of course, they are great for detox as well. Enjoy this smoothie every day and feel better, look better and be more energized.

Chapter 5: Detox Recipes For Explosive Energy

Detox is done primarily for cleansing the body by getting rid of the toxins and clearing up the digestive system. Fortunately, for those who choose to go through detox, the practice also results to additional benefits such as weight loss and an additional dose of energy. Many people have the misconception that detox is all about drinking lemon-infused water and starving for a number of days at a time. The truth of the matter is detox is about focusing on whole, fresh and healthy all-natural foods. These unprocessed foods are free from the harmful substances and toxins that many of today's junk foods are made of. More importantly, these foods are full of natural nutrients that inherently fuel the body.

One of the most powerful detox ingredients that provide explosive energy is parsley. Athletes, particularly runners who go through long distances, claim that an additional dose of parsley on any juice provides additional and explosive energy. There are those who even claim that parsley juice is so potent that one can get high by drinking it straight.

Here is a detox juice recipe that will provide explosive energy that will keep you going throughout the day.

Parsley Explosion

Ingredients:

1 cup Parsley

2 pcs. Carrots

1 pc. Apple

1 pc. Celery Stalk

Use a juicer to combine all ingredients. Start with the parsley leaves and push them in with the carrots or celery stalk. Finally, push the apple through the juicer to get the best yield. Parsley is rich in micronutrients and is known for its high amount of chlorophyll. The chlorophyll oxygenates the blood, letting it flow more easily and giving the body a boost of energy.

Green Juice Recipe

Aside from parsley, another detox vegetable that is becoming popular with fitness enthusiasts is kale. Kale is a leafy vegetable that is considered as a nutrition powerhouse because of its vitamin, mineral and nutrient content. Some of its benefits include cancer prevention, anti-inflammatory effects, lower cholesterol levels and stronger bones. Try this green juice recipe to keep you energized.

Ingredients:

2/3 cup spinach

½ cup kale

2 pcs. celery stalks

1 pc. green apple

1 pc. lime

½ inch ginger segment

Combine all ingredients using a juicer, adding a tablespoon or two of water to help create a smooth puree. The celery, apple, lime and ginger components are known for boosting the immune system, while kale and spinach are recognized for their energy-providing and cancer-fighting properties.

Chapter 6: Detox Recipes For Weight Loss

Detox as an effective way to lose weight is gaining more and more popularity all over the world. One of the main reasons why detox is an effective program for weight loss is because it focuses on the consumption of low-calorie and highly nutritious foods. On top of the decreased level of calories consumed, detox also improves your metabolism and boosts the digestive system, making it easier to shed those extra fats and weight.

Pomegranate Pineapple Lemon Juice

Weight loss does not always have to be excruciatingly filled with tasteless foods. In fact, the good thing about detox for weight loss is having the room for incorporating the tastes and ingredients that are to your personal liking. This citrusy lemon drink is balanced with the sweetness of ripe pineapples. Lemon is a well-known cleansing and detox ingredient while the water is essential for hydrating and cleansing the body. For anti-aging benefits, this also makes use of pomegranate, one of the most popular sources of antioxidants.

Ingredients:

1 cup pineapples, chopped

½ cup pomegranate juice

1 ½ cup water

½ pc/ lemon, juiced

1-inch piece ginger

Combine all ingredients except the pomegranate juice in a blender and process until it forms a smooth puree. Remove from the blender and pass through a strainer to remove any lumps. Finally, pour the pomegranate juice into the pineapple, lemon and ginger mix and stir to combine. Enjoy on a glass with ice and have a refreshing drink!

Detox Water

One of the easiest things that you can enjoy with a detox program is detox water. Simply mix your water with a few healthy ingredients and enjoy it throughout the rest of the day to enjoy the benefits. For this recipe, all you need is a water container, a knife to slice your ingredients, and some ice to make the refreshing drink even more enjoyable.

Ingredients:

½ gallon water

6 pcs. grapefruit wedges

1 pc. tangerine

½ pc. cucumber

2 pcs. peppermint or mint leaves

*ice

Wash all ingredients and prepare the fruits and vegetables by peeling the grapefruit and slicing the tangerine and cucumber. Put the ingredients in half gallon of water and let sit for at least 2hours to enjoy maximum benefits. Grapefruit aids the body's metabolic functions while cucumber keeps the body feeling full. The added mint leaves also improve the digestive process, making this drink one of the best fat-burning thirst-quenchers available today.

Chapter 7: Liver Cleanse Detox

The liver is one of the most important organs of the body, with the function of filtering dangerous toxins from the blood. As detox is known for helping to remove the same toxins from the body, it is no wonder that detox has also been found to be an effective liver cleanser. Being at the heart of removing toxins however, the liver is also one of the hardest organs to cleanse. Given a regular detox program, a liver detox and cleansing comes in only at the latter phases.

It is usual to undertake a liver cleanse after undergoing colon cleansing and kidney flushing. This phase is considered as one of the most intensive as it attempts to get rid of all the fats, poisons, old cholesterol residues, drug residues, and toxic wastes from the liver.

A 5-day liver detox is often required to achieve the aforementioned results. Most liver detox programs will consist of three juice-fast days and two raw food days. For those who can handle it, however, a 5-day juice fast is highly recommended to fully cleanse the liver and flush it of all toxins and unnecessary residues.

Morning Flush Recipe

Start with a morning flush recipe made from oranges, lemons, ginger and garlic. This recipe is recommended one hour after drinking a full glass of water in the morning. Start by having all ingredients for the whole 5-day liver detox period ready to make things easier.

Ingredients:

Whole organic oranges for juicing

5 pcs. lemons

1 bottle extra virgin olive oil

1 pc. ginger root (approximately 5 inches in length

4 pcs. garlic bulbs

Using a blender, mix together one cup of freshly squeezed orange juice, one piece lemon, also juiced, one clove of garlic, a tablespoon of olive oil, and about an inch of ginger root. Start by liquefying the ginger and garlic first, using a little bit of the orange juice to help make it easier to blend. Once the ginger and garlic have been liquefied, add in the juices and the oil. Finally, add half a cup to one cup of water. Drink this morning flush recipe every morning for 5 days of undergoing liver detox, increasing the amount of garlic by one clove every time.

Chapter 8: Migraine And Headache Detox Recipe

Relief from migraine and headache is yet another benefit that can come from detox. These stressful pains are often a result of dehydration, which is one of the issues that detox readily resolves. Also known for triggering migraine and headaches are toxins or foreign substances that can be harmful for the body. By getting rid of such toxins and harmful substances through the process of detox, migraines and headaches can be avoided altogether.

Migraine Be Gone

Green vegetables are ideal for cleansing toxins and for healing the body's systems, while other vegetables naturally hydrate the body and keep it functioning properly. This recipe contains at least three ingredients that can offer relief to migraines and headaches. That is, you can expect your headaches to tone down and even disappear once you serve yourself a glass of this migraine be gone juice.

Ingredients:

2 cups water

1 cup pineapple

1 cup kale

1 pc. celery stalk

½ pc. lemon, juiced

1 cup cucumber, cut into small slices

½ inch ginger root

1 ½ cups ice

Simple blend all ingredients in a blender and run until you have a smooth consistency. Pineapple has long been linked to easing pain and has been found to have anti-inflammatory properties, while cucumber and celery are naturally hydrating. Ginger is another anti-inflammatory ingredient that will help keep the heat and the stress down.

Chapter 9: Detox Recipes For Digestive Health

At the core of every detox diet is the commitment to enriching digestive health. Digestive health is given an added boost when the wastes and toxins are released from the body. Detox is also a healthy and natural way of keeping the body fully hydrated, making it easier for the digestive system, along with the other systems of the body, to function properly. When it comes to improving overall digestive health, you can be sure that any detox diet that successfully gets rid of the toxins in the body is what you can rely on. Here are some detox recipes for digestive health that could help you stay healthy and lose weight at the same time.

Dandelion Tea

Experts in the field of herbal medicine have found that the dandelion, a very common flowering plant, is a rich source of Vitamin A, calcium, iron and potassium. For this reason, food and drinks are sometimes enhanced with this ingredient, turning them into detox agents. The nutrients and properties of the dandelion produce a cleansing effect as it serves as a natural diuretic. It aids in the digestive process, helping the body flush out toxins and wastes through the liver and the kidneys.

Make a healthy detox dandelion tea by using 6 tablespoons of dried dandelion root and 12 tablespoons of fresh dandelion leaves. Brew the ingredients in 4 cups of boiling water for a couple of minutes. For an easier fix, you can simply crush a handful of dandelion leaves and let them brew in a cup of boiling water for about ten minutes.

Cranberry Juice

Cranberry juice is another detox ingredient that you can infuse into teas or other drinks. Even when drinking it by itself, cranberry juice already offers a load of benefits for the digestive system.

Evidence shows that cranberry juice helps in preventing urinary tract infections as well as ulcers in many individuals. On top of this, the juice is a source of vitamin C and antioxidants, making it a popular detox ingredient.

Pump up your cranberry juice by boosting it with some fiber to keep the digestive system healthy. Combine one part cranberry juice with four parts water, then add a tablespoon of apple pectin and a tablespoon of psyllium fiber. This will stimulate the intestines and help clear the digestive system in a natural and healthy manner.

Chapter 10: Detox Cleanse Step-By-Step Plan

Detox diets come in different forms. There are detox cleanse plans that can take as little as one day, while others fill the whole stretch of over 30 days. The type of detox plan will mostly depend on a person's goals and their own restrictions, but all of these options maintain the basic principles of a detox cleanse diet. If you plan to take on detox cleansing yourself, here is a simple step-by-step plan that you can use to help jumpstart the process.

Step 1: The Personal Assessment

A detox is much like anything else that a person does: it starts out with a goal and is followed by the commitment to see it through. To formulate a goal and find the dedication to see it through, you must have a clear picture of what is currently happening. This clear and present view is what should lead you to think of the things that should be happening or the changes that need to be made.

Detox is oftentimes taken on by people who, quite frankly, are unhealthy. You can go for a medical check-up and see if anything is wrong. Sometimes, even your stress levels and mood swings can be a sign that something is already wrong with your body. Sluggishness and lack of energy along with recurring pains can also be signs that there are toxins in your body that you need to flush out. Make the decision to address issues in your health and lifestyle. It is time to make a change.

Step 2: Check your Schedule

Check your schedule to see if you do have the time to perform the detoxification process. Again, a detox can be as simple as a one-day plan, or it can take up a whole month or even more. The practical mode of action would be to see if you have any occasions lined up that will cause you to eat foods restricted to a detox diet.

If this is the case, either wait for the event to be finished, or follow a cleansing plan that will be over before it. Taking a look at your schedule will give you an idea of how many days you can actually dedicate to your detox plan, thus helping you decide on a specific plan to follow. Keep in mind that undergoing the detox program can lead to withdrawal symptoms such as headaches and cravings, so be sure to consider that when choosing your detox program.

Step 3: Know what you can and can't Eat

Going through detox is a big deal, but mostly because it gets you out of your comfort zone of what you are used to eating. Here is a short list of some of the things that you can and can't eat. Make sure to keep this in mind before, during, and after your detox.

Eat	Don't Eat
Whole vegetables	Dairy and eggs
Leafy greens	Processed foods
Whole fruits	Processed sugars
Whole nuts and seeds	Coffee, soda, alcohol
Beans	Beef
Non-gluten grains	Pork
Fresh fruit juice	Whey protein

Step 4: Focus

Detox is not just about cleansing the body, but also cleansing the mind and spirituality. You may be tempted to be grumpy given all the restrictions in a detox diet, but instead of doing so, do some meditation exercises that will help you focus on inner peace and balance. Let go of stress, anger and other hateful feelings that are also filling your body with toxins. Do yoga exercises, read a book, or even go out and exercise. All the stress and negative feelings that you would have spent eating can be used for something productive. Cleanse your body and cleanse your mind and spirit as well.

Conclusion

Thank you again for purchasing the book Detox Recipes and a step-by-step plan on how to get you started!

I am extremely excited to pass this information along to you, and I am so happy that you now have read and can hopefully implement these strategies going forward.

I hope this book was able to help you understand the basics of detox and cleansing and how to use the principles to enjoy recipes that will help you cleanse your body, experience more energy and shed a few extra pounds as well.

The next step is to get started using this information and to hopefully live a more meaningful and fulfilled life!

Please don't be someone who just reads this information and doesn't apply it, the strategies in this book will only benefit you if you use them!

If you know of anyone else that could benefit from the information presented here please inform them of this book.

Finally, if you enjoyed this book and feel it has added value to your life in any way, please take the time to share your thoughts and post a review on Amazon. It'd be greatly appreciated!

Thank you and good luck!

Preview Of:

The Ayurveda Ultimate Guide!

<u>Ayurveda</u>

Ayurvedic Healing For Health, Yoga And Weight Loss, Mindful Eating, Anti-Aging And More!

Introduction

I want to thank you and congratulate you for purchasing the book, *"The Ayurveda Ultimate Guide! Ayurvedic Healing For Health, Yoga And Weight Loss, Mindful Eating, Anti-Aging And More!"*

This book contains proven steps and strategies on how to practice Ayurveda. This is a very ancient healing system, originating from the ancient Indian civilization. It has been practiced for thousands of years and has been proven to provide various health benefits.

Learn what Ayurveda is all about. In this book, you will get to know what Ayurveda specifically does in order to promote health. This practice not only keeps the body healthy, but also the mind and the spirit.

Read on and find out more about Ayurveda. Also, learn how you can achieve overall health, weight loss, and living a healthy and happy life.

Thanks again for purchasing this book, I hope you enjoy it!

Chapter 1: Understanding Ayurveda

Ayurveda is an ancient traditional healing practice. It uses the holistic or "whole body" healing system. The practice originated from the ancient Indian civilization.

The practice stems from the belief that health is achieved through maintaining harmony between the body, spirit, and mind. Creating and maintaining the balance is a delicate process that determines wellness and health.

Concepts in Ayurveda

Ayurveda revolves around the theory that everything that exists in the universe is connected to each other. Existence is in harmony with the rest of the universe.

Within the body, this same harmony should also exist in order to achieve good health. There should be harmony between the mind and body, as well as the spirit. These 3 elements should also be in harmony with the rest of the universe. Disruption in the balance causes sickness and poor health.

Ayurveda is firmly based on the concept that the spirit, body and mind are all connected. Maintaining the balance is the most important focus of Ayurveda. The basic tenets of Ayurveda based on this central concept are:

- All things are connected, whether living or nonliving things. Each thing contains the same basic 5 elements of earth, air, water, space, and fire.

- The body and the environment have a deep connection.

- There is a connection from the body, to the people around it, to its immediate environment, and to the rest of the universe. Balance among these supports good health.

- Health is retained if the balance is maintained, through wholesome, effective interaction with the environment.

- The initial balance is often disrupted by the lifestyle one leads. Choices in profession, relationships, diet, and exercise creates imbalances in the physical, spiritual, and emotional aspects.

- Imbalance disrupts harmony and invites diseases.

- Restoring and maintaining balance is a conscious act. Each person has the responsibility to take steps in achieving harmony within the self and with the environment.

Anything can disrupt the balance by affecting the emotional, physical and spiritual well-being. Some of those that can cause disruption include:

- injuries
- emotional stress
- genetic or birth defects
- age
- climate and seasonal changes

In Ayurveda, people have the 5 basic elements of the universe within them. These are:

- space: related to expansiveness
- fire: related to heat, fire and transformation

- air: related to mobility, lack of form and gaseousness
- earth: related to stability and solidity
- water: related to instability and liquidity

In the body, these elements combine to form the doshas, the life energies or forces. These doshas work together and control how the body functions. There are 3 doshas working in the body, namely:

- vatadosha (combination of the element of air and space)
- kaphadosha (earth and water)
- pitta dosha (water and fire)

The Doshas

The doshas are inherited. The mix of doshas in each person is unique. Most often, one dosha appears to be more dominant over the others. Each of the doshas has specific body functions to control. Imbalance in the doshas and in their functions is held in Ayurveda as one of the factors that determine sickness and health.

Vatadosha

Vatadosha is the combination of air and space. This is considered in Ayurveda as the most powerful of the three doshas. The vatadosha controls the basic body functions like cellular division. Vatadosha is considered as the moving force behind the kaphadosha and the pitta dosha. The center of this energy is in the colon. It balances emotion and thoughts. It also supports activity, clear comprehension, and creativity.

A person with a dominant vatadosha tends to be restless, alert, and quick. They are also fearful, anxious and nervous. These people are at higher risk for the following health problems:

- constipation
- arthritis
- flatulence
- insomnia
- nerve disorders

Balancing vata includes avoidance of extreme temperatures, maintaining calm and routine, and getting adequate rest. The energy of vata increases as one ages.

Vata controls the following functions:

- breathing
- mind
- heart function
- blood flow
- excretion via the intestines

There are things that can affect the vatadosha and disrupt its normal function, such as the following:

- grief
- fear
- eating dry fruit
- staying up late
- inadequate time in between meals

Disruptions in the vatadosha can increase the risk of developing the following health problems:

- anxious feelings
- asthma attacks
- cardiovascular disease

- disorders of the nervous system
- rheumatoid arthritis
- skin irritations

Pitta dosha

The pitta dosha is a combination of the elements of water and fire. Pitta dosha regulates the chemical, digestive, and metabolic functions. It is often associated with oiliness and heat. The center of this energy is the small intestines.

Energy from the pitta dosha adds a healthy glow to the skin, eyes, and hair. It controls the following bodily functions:

- digestion
- metabolic processes to break down ingested foods
- hormones that control appetite

Dominance of this dosha supports a hearty appetite and efficient metabolism. People with this dosha dominance tend to be aggressive and intelligent achievers.

In terms of health, the dominance of pitta dosha makes a person prone to the following health problems:

- nausea and vomiting
- inflammatory conditions
- rashes
- diarrhea
- bleeding disorders
- anger

Balance is achieved by avoiding exposure to extreme heat and limiting eating spicy food.

The pitta dosha can be disrupted by the following:

- fatigue
- eating foods that are spicy
- eating foods that are sour
- too much exposure to the sun

Disruptions in the pitta dosha increase the risk for the development of the following health problems:

- heart disease
- high blood pressure
- anger
- negative emotions
- infections
- Crohn's disease
- heartburn (often a few hours after eating)

Kaphadosha

This dosha is composed of the elements of earth and water. It controls the following bodily functions:

- growth of muscles
- weight
- stability and strength
- immune system

Factors that can disrupt the kaphadosha include the following:

- sleeping during the day
- greed
- eating even after the stomach is already full
- eating lots of sweet foods
- too much intake of salt or water

Imbalance in the kaphadosha increases the chances of a person suffering from the following:

- asthma and other respiratory disorders
- diabetes
- cancer
- obesity
- nausea, often experienced a few minutes after eating

The seat or center of kapha is in the stomach. It is related to all things that involve mucus and lubrication. It is also related to the arterial system as well as the immune system.

According to Ayurveda, the kaphadosha produces energy that promotes healing and self-repair. It allows for endurance. Energy from kaphadosha provides psychological and physical stability and strength. In terms of emotions, it promotes patience, understanding, empathy, forgiveness, compassion, love and loyalty.

People with dominant kapha have strong personalities. They are loving and are known to be tolerant. They are also tenacious, but can keep calm at the same time.

In as far as health is concerned; the dominance of kapha energy makes a person naturally prone to the following problems:

- lethargy
- weight gain
- goiter
- excessive sleep
- pulmonary congestion
- asthma
- allergies

Health maintenance is achieved through regular exercise, avoidance of napping, and eating light meals.

Thanks for Previewing My Exciting Book Entitled:

"Ayurveda: The Ayurveda Ultimate Guide! Ayurvedic Healing For Health, Yoga And Weight Loss, Mindful Eating, Anti-Aging And More!"

To purchase this book, simply go to the Amazon Kindle store and simply search:

"AYURVEDA"

Then just scroll down until you see my book. You will know it is mine because you will see my name "Sarah Brooks" underneath the title.

Alternatively, you can visit my author page on Amazon to see this book and other work I have done. Thanks so much, and please don't forget your free bonuses

DON'T LEAVE YET! - CHECK OUT YOUR FREE BONUSES BELOW!

Free Bonus Offer: Get Free Access To The LiveFitVIP.com VIP Newsletter!

Once you enter your email address you will immediately get free access to this awesome newsletter!

But wait, right now if you join now for free you will also get free access to the "The 7 Keys To Body Transformation" free EBook!

To claim both your FREE VIP NEWSLETTER MEMBERSHIP and your FREE BONUS EBook on THE 7 KEYS TO BODY TRANSFORMATION!

Just Go To:

www.liveFitVIP.com